FOOD *AND* EXERCISE JOURNAL

TRAIN.
EAT.
SLEEP.
REPEAT.

MY NAME

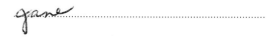

....

ISBN-13: 978-1546386612
ISBN-10: 1546386610

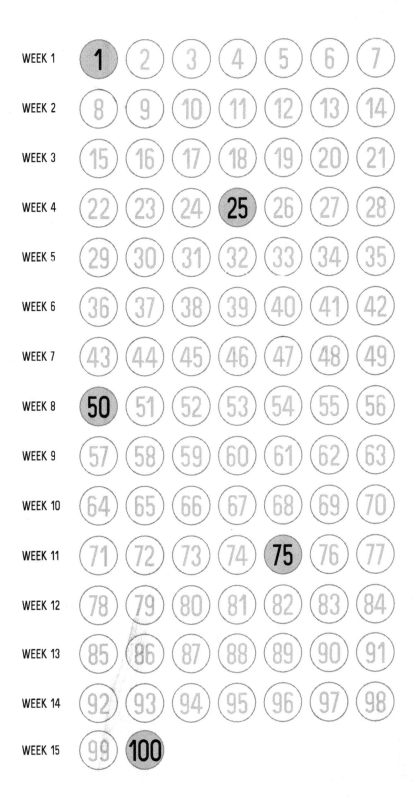

HOW I FEEL

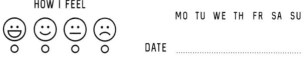

MO TU WE TH FR SA SU

DATE ....

DAY 20

BREAKFAST	LUNCH	DINNER
....	....	....
....	....	....
....	....	....
....	....	....
....	....	....

SNACKS

....

....

....

TOTAL CALORIES

WEIGHT   SLEEP   WATER   PROTEIN

OTHER

....

EXERCISE / OTHER ACTIVITIES	SET / REPS / DISTANCE	TIME
....	....	....
....	....	....
....	....	....
....	....	....
....	....	....

NOTES

....

....

....

6A   7   8   9   10   11   12P   1   2   3   4   5   6   7   8   9   10+

B=BREAKFAST   L=LUNCH   D=DINNER   S=SNACKS   E=EXERCISE

DAY (21)

DATE ....

HOW I FEEL

😀 ○ 😊 ○ 😐 ○ ☹ ○

BREAKFAST	LUNCH	DINNER
....	....	....
....	....	....
....	....	....
....	....	....
....	....	....

SNACKS

....
....
....

TOTAL CALORIES

OTHER

....

WEIGHT **SLEEP** **WATER** **PROTEIN**

♥ EXERCISE / OTHER ACTIVITIES   SET / REPS / DISTANCE   TIME

....	....	....
....	....	....
....	....	....
....	....	....
....	....	....

NOTES

....
....
....

🕐 6A 7 8 9 10 11 12P 1 2 3 4 5 6 7 8 9 10+

B=BREAKFAST   L=LUNCH   D=DINNER   S=SNACKS   E=EXERCISE

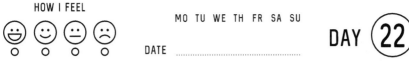

HOW I FEEL

MO TU WE TH FR SA SU

DATE ....

DAY (22)

BREAKFAST   LUNCH   DINNER

SNACKS

TOTAL CALORIES

WEIGHT   SLEEP   WATER   PROTEIN

OTHER

EXERCISE / OTHER ACTIVITIES   SET / REPS / DISTANCE   TIME

NOTES

6A   7   8   9   10   11   12P   1   2   3   4   5   6   7   8   9   10+

B=BREAKFAST   L=LUNCH   D=DINNER   S=SNACKS   E=EXERCISE

DAY (23)

MO TU WE TH FR SA SU

DATE ....

😃 ◯ 🙂 ◯ 😐 ◯ 🙁 ◯

BREAKFAST	LUNCH	DINNER
....	....	....
....	....	....
....	....	....
....	....	....
....	....	....

SNACKS

TOTAL CALORIES

WEIGHT   SLEEP   WATER   PROTEIN

OTHER

....

❤ EXERCISE / OTHER ACTIVITIES   SET / REPS / DISTANCE   TIME

NOTES

....

....

....

🕐 6A 7 8 9 10 11 12P 1 2 3 4 5 6 7 8 9 10+

B=BREAKFAST L=LUNCH D=DINNER S=SNACKS E=EXERCISE

HOW I FEEL

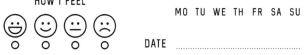

😀 ☺ 😐 ☹
○ ○ ○ ○

MO TU WE TH FR SA SU

DATE ....

DAY (24)

BREAKFAST	LUNCH	DINNER

SNACKS

TOTAL CALORIES

OTHER

WEIGHT   SLEEP   WATER   PROTEIN

....

❤ EXERCISE / OTHER ACTIVITIES   SET / REPS / DISTANCE   TIME

NOTES

....

....

....

🕐 6A 7 8 9 10 11 12P 1 2 3 4 5 6 7 8 9 10+

B=BREAKFAST L=LUNCH D=DINNER S=SNACKS E=EXERCISE

DAY (25)

DATE ....

HOW I FEEL

😀 ○   🙂 ○   😐 ○   🙁 ○

BREAKFAST   LUNCH   DINNER

....
....
....
....
....

SNACKS

....
....
....

TOTAL CALORIES

WEIGHT   SLEEP   WATER   PROTEIN

OTHER

....

❤ EXERCISE / OTHER ACTIVITIES   SET / REPS / DISTANCE   TIME

....
....
....
....
....

NOTES

....
....
....

🕐   6A 7 8 9 10 11 12P 1 2 3 4 5 6 7 8 9 10+

B=BREAKFAST   L=LUNCH   D=DINNER   S=SNACKS   E=EXERCISE

DAY 25

MY MEASUREMENTS

[1] NECK

[2] CHEST

[3] ARMS

[4] WAIST

[5] ABDOMEN

[6] HIPS

[7] THIGHS

[8] CALVES

WEIGHT

BMI

DAY (26)

MO TU WE TH FR SA SU

DATE ....

BREAKFAST   LUNCH   DINNER

.... | .... | ....
.... | .... | ....
.... | .... | ....
.... | .... | ....
.... | .... | ....

SNACKS

.... | .... | ....
.... | .... | ....
.... | .... | ....

TOTAL CALORIES

===================

OTHER

          WEIGHT   SLEEP   WATER   PROTEIN

....

EXERCISE / OTHER ACTIVITIES   SET / REPS / DISTANCE   TIME

.... | .... | ....
.... | .... | ....
.... | .... | ....
.... | .... | ....
.... | .... | ....

NOTES

....
....
....

6A 7 8 9 10 11 12P 1 2 3 4 5 6 7 8 9 10+

B=BREAKFAST   L=LUNCH   D=DINNER   S=SNACKS   E=EXERCISE

HOW I FEEL

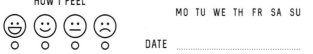

MO TU WE TH FR SA SU

DATE ....

DAY (27)

BREAKFAST   LUNCH   DINNER

SNACKS

TOTAL CALORIES

OTHER

WEIGHT   SLEEP   WATER   PROTEIN

EXERCISE / OTHER ACTIVITIES   SET / REPS / DISTANCE   TIME

NOTES

6A   7   8   9   10   11   12P   1   2   3   4   5   6   7   8   9   10+

B=BREAKFAST   L=LUNCH   D=DINNER   S=SNACKS   E=EXERCISE

DAY (28)

MO TU WE TH FR SA SU

DATE ....

HOW I FEEL

BREAKFAST · LUNCH · DINNER

....
....
....
....
....

SNACKS

TOTAL CALORIES

WEIGHT · SLEEP · WATER · PROTEIN

OTHER

....

EXERCISE / OTHER ACTIVITIES · SET / REPS / DISTANCE · TIME

NOTES

....
....
....

6A 7 8 9 10 11 12P 1 2 3 4 5 6 7 8 9 10+

B=BREAKFAST   L=LUNCH   D=DINNER   S=SNACKS   E=EXERCISE

HOW I FEEL

MO TU WE TH FR SA SU

DATE ....

DAY (29)

BREAKFAST	LUNCH	DINNER
....	....	....
....	....	....
....	....	....
....	....	....
....	....	....

SNACKS

....

....

....

TOTAL CALORIES

WEIGHT   SLEEP   WATER   PROTEIN

OTHER

....

EXERCISE / OTHER ACTIVITIES   SET / REPS / DISTANCE   TIME

....	....	....
....	....	....
....	....	....
....	....	....
....	....	....

NOTES

....

....

....

6A   7   8   9   10   11   12P   1   2   3   4   5   6   7   8   9   10+

B=BREAKFAST   L=LUNCH   D=DINNER   S=SNACKS   E=EXERCISE

DAY (30)

MO TU WE TH FR SA SU

DATE ....

HOW I FEEL

😀 🙂 😐 🙁
○ ○ ○ ○

BREAKFAST   LUNCH   DINNER

....
....
....
....
....

SNACKS   ....
....
....
....

TOTAL CALORIES

WEIGHT   SLEEP   WATER   PROTEIN

OTHER

....

 EXERCISE / OTHER ACTIVITIES   SET / REPS / DISTANCE   TIME

....
....
....
....
....

NOTES

....
....
....

6A 7 8 9 10 11 12P 1 2 3 4 5 6 7 8 9 10+

B=BREAKFAST   L=LUNCH   D=DINNER   S=SNACKS   E=EXERCISE

HOW I FEEL

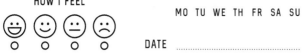

MO TU WE TH FR SA SU

DATE ....

DAY (31)

BREAKFAST   LUNCH   DINNER

....
....
....
....
....

SNACKS

....
....
....
....

TOTAL CALORIES

OTHER   WEIGHT   SLEEP   WATER   PROTEIN

....

EXERCISE / OTHER ACTIVITIES   SET / REPS / DISTANCE   TIME

....
....
....
....
....

NOTES

....
....
....

6A 7 8 9 10 11 12P 1 2 3 4 5 6 7 8 9 10+

B=BREAKFAST   L=LUNCH   D=DINNER   S=SNACKS   E=EXERCISE

DAY (32)

MO TU WE TH FR SA SU

DATE ....

HOW I FEEL

BREAKFAST

LUNCH

DINNER

SNACKS

TOTAL CALORIES

OTHER

WEIGHT   SLEEP   WATER   PROTEIN

♡ **EXERCISE / OTHER ACTIVITIES**   SET / REPS / DISTANCE   TIME

NOTES

6A 7 8 9 10 11 12P 1 2 3 4 5 6 7 8 9 10+

B=BREAKFAST   L=LUNCH   D=DINNER   S=SNACKS   E=EXERCISE

HOW I FEEL

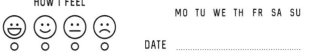

MO TU WE TH FR SA SU

DATE ....

DAY 33

BREAKFAST | LUNCH | DINNER

SNACKS

TOTAL CALORIES

OTHER

....

WEIGHT   SLEEP   WATER   PROTEIN

EXERCISE / OTHER ACTIVITIES   SET / REPS / DISTANCE   TIME

NOTES

....
....
....

6A 7 8 9 10 11 12P 1 2 3 4 5 6 7 8 9 10+

B=BREAKFAST L=LUNCH D=DINNER S=SNACKS E=EXERCISE

DAY (34)

MO TU WE TH FR SA SU

DATE ....

HOW I FEEL

😃 ☺ 😐 ☹
○ ○ ○ ○

BREAKFAST

LUNCH

DINNER

SNACKS

TOTAL CALORIES

WEIGHT   SLEEP   WATER   PROTEIN

OTHER

....

♡ EXERCISE / OTHER ACTIVITIES

SET / REPS / DISTANCE   TIME

NOTES

....
....
....

6A 7 8 9 10 11 12P 1 2 3 4 5 6 7 8 9 10+

B=BREAKFAST   L=LUNCH   D=DINNER   S=SNACKS   E=EXERCISE

HOW I FEEL

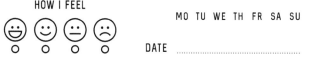

MO TU WE TH FR SA SU

DATE ....

DAY (35)

BREAKFAST   LUNCH   DINNER

....
....
....
....
....

SNACKS   ....
....
....
....

TOTAL CALORIES

OTHER   WEIGHT   SLEEP   WATER   PROTEIN

....

EXERCISE / OTHER ACTIVITIES   SET / REPS / DISTANCE   TIME

....
....
....
....
....

NOTES
....
....
....

6A 7 8 9 10 11 12P 1 2 3 4 5 6 7 8 9 10+
B=BREAKFAST   L=LUNCH   D=DINNER   S=SNACKS   E=EXERCISE

DAY (36)

DATE ....

HOW I FEEL

😃 🙂 😐 🙁
○ ○ ○ ○

BREAKFAST   LUNCH   DINNER

....
....
....
....
....
_____ ____   ....

SNACKS   ....
....
....
....
_____ ____ _____ ____ _____ ____

TOTAL CALORIES

WEIGHT   SLEEP   WATER   PROTEIN

_____

OTHER

....

💓 EXERCISE / OTHER ACTIVITIES   SET / REPS / DISTANCE   TIME

....
....
....
....
....
_____   _____   _____

NOTES

....
....
....

🕐 6A 7 8 9 10 11 12P 1 2 3 4 5 6 7 8 9 10+

B=BREAKFAST   L=LUNCH   D=DINNER   S=SNACKS   E=EXERCISE

HOW I FEEL

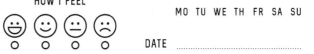

☺ ☺ ☺ ☺
○ ○ ○ ○

MO TU WE TH FR SA SU

DATE ....

DAY (37)

BREAKFAST   LUNCH   DINNER

....
....
....
....
....
_____ ____   ....

SNACKS   ....
....
....
....
_____ ____ _____ ____ _____ ____

TOTAL CALORIES
_____   WEIGHT   SLEEP   WATER   PROTEIN
OTHER
....

EXERCISE / OTHER ACTIVITIES   SET / REPS / DISTANCE   TIME

....
....
....
....
....
_____   _____   _____

NOTES
....
....
....

6A   7   8   9   10   11   12P   1   2   3   4   5   6   7   8   9   10+
B=BREAKFAST   L=LUNCH   D=DINNER   S=SNACKS   E=EXERCISE

DAY (38)

MO TU WE TH FR SA SU

DATE ....

HOW I FEEL

😃 ◯ 🙂 ◯ 😐 ◯ 🙁 ◯

BREAKFAST   LUNCH   DINNER

....
....
....
....
....

SNACKS
....
....
....
....

TOTAL CALORIES

OTHER

WEIGHT   SLEEP   WATER   PROTEIN

....

♥ EXERCISE / OTHER ACTIVITIES   SET / REPS / DISTANCE   TIME

....
....
....
....
....

NOTES
....
....
....

🕐 6A 7 8 9 10 11 12P 1 2 3 4 5 6 7 8 9 10+

B=BREAKFAST L=LUNCH D=DINNER S=SNACKS E=EXERCISE

HOW I FEEL

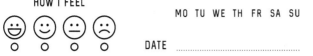

MO TU WE TH FR SA SU

DATE ....

DAY (39)

BREAKFAST   LUNCH   DINNER

SNACKS

TOTAL CALORIES

WEIGHT   SLEEP   WATER   PROTEIN

OTHER

EXERCISE / OTHER ACTIVITIES   SET / REPS / DISTANCE   TIME

NOTES

6A 7 8 9 10 11 12P 1 2 3 4 5 6 7 8 9 10+

B=BREAKFAST L=LUNCH D=DINNER S=SNACKS E=EXERCISE

DAY (40)

DATE ....

HOW I FEEL

☺ ☺ ☺ ☹
○ ○ ○ ○

BREAKFAST | LUNCH | DINNER

....
....
....
....
....

SNACKS

....
....
....

TOTAL CALORIES

OTHER

WEIGHT | SLEEP | WATER | PROTEIN

....

EXERCISE / OTHER ACTIVITIES | SET / REPS / DISTANCE | TIME

....
....
....
....
....

NOTES

....
....
....

6A 7 8 9 10 11 12P 1 2 3 4 5 6 7 8 9 10+

B=BREAKFAST   L=LUNCH   D=DINNER   S=SNACKS   E=EXERCISE

HOW I FEEL

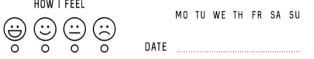

MO TU WE TH FR SA SU

DATE ....

DAY (41)

BREAKFAST   LUNCH   DINNER

....
....
....
....
....

SNACKS   ....

....
....
....

TOTAL CALORIES

WEIGHT   SLEEP   WATER   PROTEIN

OTHER

....

EXERCISE / OTHER ACTIVITIES   SET / REPS / DISTANCE   TIME

....
....
....
....
....

NOTES

....
....
....

6A 7 8 9 10 11 12P 1 2 3 4 5 6 7 8 9 10+

B=BREAKFAST   L=LUNCH   D=DINNER   S=SNACKS   E=EXERCISE

DAY (42)

MO TU WE TH FR SA SU

DATE ....

HOW I FEEL

☺ ☺ ☺ ☹
○ ○ ○ ○

BREAKFAST   LUNCH   DINNER

....
....
....
....
....

SNACKS

....
....
....

TOTAL CALORIES

WEIGHT   SLEEP   WATER   PROTEIN

OTHER

....

♥ EXERCISE / OTHER ACTIVITIES   SET / REPS / DISTANCE   TIME

....
....
....
....
....

NOTES

....
....
....

🕐 6A 7 8 9 10 11 12P 1 2 3 4 5 6 7 8 9 10+

B=BREAKFAST   L=LUNCH   D=DINNER   S=SNACKS   E=EXERCISE

HOW I FEEL

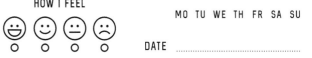

MO TU WE TH FR SA SU

DATE ....

DAY 43

BREAKFAST   LUNCH   DINNER

SNACKS

TOTAL CALORIES

OTHER

WEIGHT   SLEEP   WATER   PROTEIN

EXERCISE / OTHER ACTIVITIES   SET / REPS / DISTANCE   TIME

NOTES

6A 7 8 9 10 11 12P 1 2 3 4 5 6 7 8 9 10+

B=BREAKFAST   L=LUNCH   D=DINNER   S=SNACKS   E=EXERCISE

DAY (44)

MO TU WE TH FR SA SU

DATE ....

BREAKFAST

LUNCH

DINNER

SNACKS

TOTAL CALORIES

WEIGHT   SLEEP   WATER   PROTEIN

OTHER

EXERCISE / OTHER ACTIVITIES

SET / REPS / DISTANCE   TIME

NOTES

6A 7 8 9 10 11 12P 1 2 3 4 5 6 7 8 9 10+

B=BREAKFAST   L=LUNCH   D=DINNER   S=SNACKS   E=EXERCISE

HOW I FEEL

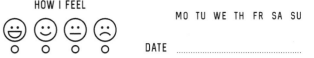

MO TU WE TH FR SA SU

DATE ....

DAY (45)

BREAKFAST   LUNCH   DINNER

SNACKS

TOTAL CALORIES

WEIGHT   SLEEP   WATER   PROTEIN

OTHER

EXERCISE / OTHER ACTIVITIES   SET / REPS / DISTANCE   TIME

NOTES

6A 7 8 9 10 11 12P 1 2 3 4 5 6 7 8 9 10+

B=BREAKFAST   L=LUNCH   D=DINNER   S=SNACKS   E=EXERCISE

DAY (46)

DATE ....

HOW I FEEL

○   ○   ○   ○

BREAKFAST   LUNCH   DINNER

....
....
....
....
....
_____ ____   ....

SNACKS   ....

....
....
....
_____ ____   _____ ____   _____ ____

TOTAL CALORIES

_____

OTHER   WEIGHT   SLEEP   WATER   PROTEIN

....

EXERCISE / OTHER ACTIVITIES   SET / REPS / DISTANCE   TIME

....
....
....
....
....
_____   _____   _____

NOTES

....
....
....

6A   7   8   9   10   11   12P   1   2   3   4   5   6   7   8   9   10+
B=BREAKFAST   L=LUNCH   D=DINNER   S=SNACKS   E=EXERCISE

HOW I FEEL

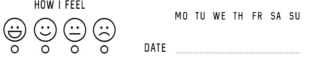

MO TU WE TH FR SA SU

DATE ....

DAY 47

BREAKFAST	LUNCH	DINNER

SNACKS

TOTAL CALORIES

WEIGHT

SLEEP

WATER

PROTEIN

OTHER

....

EXERCISE / OTHER ACTIVITIES   SET / REPS / DISTANCE   TIME

NOTES

6A 7 8 9 10 11 12P 1 2 3 4 5 6 7 8 9 10+

B=BREAKFAST L=LUNCH D=DINNER S=SNACKS E=EXERCISE

DAY (48)

DATE ....

HOW I FEEL

:D :) :| :(
O   O   O   O

BREAKFAST   LUNCH   DINNER

....
....
....
....
....

SNACKS
....
....
....

TOTAL CALORIES

WEIGHT   SLEEP   WATER   PROTEIN

OTHER
....

EXERCISE / OTHER ACTIVITIES   SET / REPS / DISTANCE   TIME

....
....
....
....
....

NOTES
....
....
....

6A 7 8 9 10 11 12P 1 2 3 4 5 6 7 8 9 10+

B=BREAKFAST   L=LUNCH   D=DINNER   S=SNACKS   E=EXERCISE

HOW I FEEL

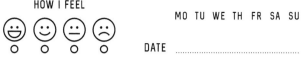

MO TU WE TH FR SA SU

DATE ....

DAY (49)

BREAKFAST   LUNCH   DINNER

....
....
....
....
....

SNACKS   ....
                             ....
....
....

TOTAL CALORIES

WEIGHT   SLEEP   WATER   PROTEIN

OTHER

....

EXERCISE / OTHER ACTIVITIES   SET / REPS / DISTANCE   TIME

....
....
....
....
....

NOTES

....
....
....

6A 7 8 9 10 11 12P 1 2 3 4 5 6 7 8 9 10+

B=BREAKFAST   L=LUNCH   D=DINNER   S=SNACKS   E=EXERCISE

DAY (50)

MO TU WE TH FR SA SU

DATE ....

HOW I FEEL

☺ ☺ ☺ ☹
○   ○   ○   ○

BREAKFAST

....
....
....
....
....

SNACKS

....
....
....

TOTAL CALORIES

OTHER

....

LUNCH

....
....
....
....
....
....
....
....
....

DINNER

....
....
....
....
....
....
....
....
....

WEIGHT   SLEEP   WATER   PROTEIN

....

♡ EXERCISE / OTHER ACTIVITIES

SET / REPS / DISTANCE   TIME

....
....
....
....
....

NOTES

....
....
....

6A 7 8 9 10 11 12P 1 2 3 4 5 6 7 8 9 10+

B=BREAKFAST L=LUNCH D=DINNER S=SNACKS E=EXERCISE

DAY 50

MY MEASUREMENTS

[1] NECK

[2] CHEST

[3] ARMS

[4] WAIST

[5] ABDOMEN

[6] HIPS

[7] THIGHS

[8] CALVES

WEIGHT

BMI

DAY (51)

MO TU WE TH FR SA SU

DATE ....

HOW I FEEL

☺ ☺ ☺ ☹
○ ○ ○ ○

BREAKFAST   LUNCH   DINNER

....
....
....
....
....

SNACKS

....
....
....

TOTAL CALORIES

WEIGHT   SLEEP   WATER   PROTEIN

OTHER

....

♥ EXERCISE / OTHER ACTIVITIES   SET / REPS / DISTANCE   TIME

....
....
....
....
....

NOTES

....
....
....

🕐 6A 7 8 9 10 11 12P 1 2 3 4 5 6 7 8 9 10+

B=BREAKFAST   L=LUNCH   D=DINNER   S=SNACKS   E=EXERCISE

HOW I FEEL

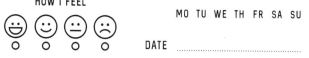

MO TU WE TH FR SA SU

DATE ....

DAY (52)

BREAKFAST   LUNCH   DINNER

SNACKS

TOTAL CALORIES

WEIGHT   SLEEP   WATER   PROTEIN

OTHER

EXERCISE / OTHER ACTIVITIES   SET / REPS / DISTANCE   TIME

NOTES

6A   7   8   9   10   11   12P   1   2   3   4   5   6   7   8   9   10+

B=BREAKFAST   L=LUNCH   D=DINNER   S=SNACKS   E=EXERCISE

DAY (53)

MO TU WE TH FR SA SU

DATE ....

BREAKFAST

....
....
....
....
....
_____   ___

SNACKS

....
....
....
_____   ___

LUNCH

....
....
....
....
....
....
....
....
....
....
....
....
....

DINNER

....
....
....
....
....
....
....
....
....
....
....

TOTAL CALORIES
_____
_____

OTHER
....

WEIGHT	SLEEP	WATER	PROTEIN

....

♥ EXERCISE / OTHER ACTIVITIES   SET / REPS / DISTANCE   TIME

....
....
....
....
....
_____   ___   ___

NOTES

....
....
....

🕐 6A 7 8 9 10 11 12P 1 2 3 4 5 6 7 8 9 10+

B=BREAKFAST L=LUNCH D=DINNER S=SNACKS E=EXERCISE

HOW I FEEL

MO TU WE TH FR SA SU

DATE ....

DAY (54)

BREAKFAST

LUNCH

DINNER

SNACKS

TOTAL CALORIES

WEIGHT   SLEEP   WATER   PROTEIN

OTHER

EXERCISE / OTHER ACTIVITIES   SET / REPS / DISTANCE   TIME

NOTES

6A 7 8 9 10 11 12P 1 2 3 4 5 6 7 8 9 10+

B=BREAKFAST   L=LUNCH   D=DINNER   S=SNACKS   E=EXERCISE

DAY (55)

MO TU WE TH FR SA SU

DATE ....

HOW I FEEL

😃 ○   🙂 ○   😐 ○   ☹ ○

BREAKFAST

....
....
....
....
....

SNACKS

....
....
....

LUNCH

....
....
....
....
....
....
....
....
....

DINNER

....
....
....
....
....
....
....
....

TOTAL CALORIES

OTHER

....

WEIGHT	SLEEP	WATER	PROTEIN

EXERCISE / OTHER ACTIVITIES

	SET / REPS / DISTANCE	TIME
....	....	....
....	....	....
....	....	....
....	....	....
....	....	....

NOTES

....
....
....

6A	7	8	9	10	11	12P	1	2	3	4	5	6	7	8	9	10+

B=BREAKFAST   L=LUNCH   D=DINNER   S=SNACKS   E=EXERCISE

HOW I FEEL

MO TU WE TH FR SA SU

DATE ....

DAY (56)

BREAKFAST   LUNCH   DINNER

....
....
....
....
....

SNACKS   ....
                          ....
....
....
....

TOTAL CALORIES

WEIGHT   SLEEP   WATER   PROTEIN

OTHER

....

EXERCISE / OTHER ACTIVITIES   SET / REPS / DISTANCE   TIME

....
....
....
....
....

NOTES

....
....
....

6A 7   8   9   10 11 12P 1   2   3   4   5   6   7   8   9   10+
B=BREAKFAST   L=LUNCH   D=DINNER   S=SNACKS   E=EXERCISE

DAY (57)

DATE ....

HOW I FEEL

😃 ◯   🙂 ◯   😐 ◯   🙁 ◯

BREAKFAST

....
....
....
....
....
_____

SNACKS

....
....
....

TOTAL CALORIES

═══════════════

LUNCH

....
....
....
....
....
....
....
....

DINNER

....
....
....
....
....
....
....
....

WEIGHT   SLEEP   WATER   PROTEIN

OTHER

....

EXERCISE / OTHER ACTIVITIES	SET / REPS / DISTANCE	TIME
....	....	....
....	....	....
....	....	....
....	....	....
....	....	....

NOTES

....
....
....

6A   7   8   9   10   11   12P   1   2   3   4   5   6   7   8   9   10+

B=BREAKFAST   L=LUNCH   D=DINNER   S=SNACKS   E=EXERCISE

HOW I FEEL

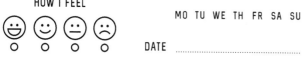

MO TU WE TH FR SA SU

DATE ....

DAY (58)

BREAKFAST	LUNCH	DINNER

SNACKS

TOTAL CALORIES

OTHER

WEIGHT **SLEEP** **WATER** **PROTEIN**

EXERCISE / OTHER ACTIVITIES   SET / REPS / DISTANCE   TIME

NOTES

6A 7 8 9 10 11 12P 1 2 3 4 5 6 7 8 9 10+

B=BREAKFAST L=LUNCH D=DINNER S=SNACKS E=EXERCISE

DAY (59)

DATE ....

HOW I FEEL

😀 ○   🙂 ○   😐 ○   🙁 ○

BREAKFAST

....
....
....
....
....

SNACKS

....
....
....

LUNCH

....
....
....
....
....
....
....
....
....
....
....

DINNER

....
....
....
....
....

TOTAL CALORIES

OTHER

....

WEIGHT	SLEEP	WATER	PROTEIN

....

EXERCISE / OTHER ACTIVITIES

	SET / REPS / DISTANCE	TIME
....	....	....
....	....	....
....	....	....
....	....	....
....	....	....

NOTES

....
....
....

6A	7	8	9	10	11	12P	1	2	3	4	5	6	7	8	9	10+

B=BREAKFAST   L=LUNCH   D=DINNER   S=SNACKS   E=EXERCISE

HOW I FEEL

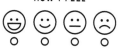

MO TU WE TH FR SA SU

DATE ....

DAY (60)

BREAKFAST   LUNCH   DINNER

....
....
....
....
....
                         ....
SNACKS   ....
                         ....
....
....
....

TOTAL CALORIES

WEIGHT   SLEEP   WATER   PROTEIN

OTHER

....

EXERCISE / OTHER ACTIVITIES   SET / REPS / DISTANCE   TIME

....
....
....
....
....

NOTES

....
....
....

    6A   7   8   9   10   11   12P   1   2   3   4   5   6   7   8   9   10+
....

B=BREAKFAST   L=LUNCH   D=DINNER   S=SNACKS   E=EXERCISE

DAY (61)

MO TU WE TH FR SA SU

DATE ....

HOW I FEEL

:D :) :| :(
O   O   O   O

BREAKFAST   LUNCH   DINNER

....
....
....
....
....

SNACKS
                   ....
....
....
....

TOTAL CALORIES

WEIGHT   SLEEP   WATER   PROTEIN

OTHER

....

EXERCISE / OTHER ACTIVITIES   SET / REPS / DISTANCE   TIME

....
....
....
....
....

NOTES

....
....
....

6A   7   8   9   10   11   12P   1   2   3   4   5   6   7   8   9   10+
B=BREAKFAST   L=LUNCH   D=DINNER   S=SNACKS   E=EXERCISE

HOW I FEEL

MO TU WE TH FR SA SU

DATE ....

DAY (62)

BREAKFAST

....
....
....
....
....

SNACKS

....
....
....

TOTAL CALORIES

OTHER
....

LUNCH

....
....
....
....
....
....
....
....
....

DINNER

....
....
....
....
....

WEIGHT   SLEEP   WATER   PROTEIN

....

EXERCISE / OTHER ACTIVITIES

EXERCISE / OTHER ACTIVITIES	SET / REPS / DISTANCE	TIME
....	....	....
....	....	....
....	....	....
....	....	....
....	....	....

NOTES

....
....
....

 6A 7 8 9 10 11 12P 1 2 3 4 5 6 7 8 9 10+

B=BREAKFAST L=LUNCH D=DINNER S=SNACKS E=EXERCISE

DAY (63)

MO TU WE TH FR SA SU

DATE ....

HOW I FEEL

☺ ☺ ☺ ☹
○ ○ ○ ○

BREAKFAST

....
....
....
....
....

SNACKS

....
....
....

TOTAL CALORIES

OTHER

....

LUNCH

....
....
....
....
....
....
....
....
....

DINNER

....
....
....
....
....
....
....
....
....

WEIGHT   **SLEEP**   **WATER**   **PROTEIN**

....

❤ **EXERCISE / OTHER ACTIVITIES**   SET / REPS / DISTANCE   TIME

....
....
....
....
....
....

NOTES

....
....
....

🕐 6A 7 8 9 10 11 12P 1 2 3 4 5 6 7 8 9 10+
B=BREAKFAST   L=LUNCH   D=DINNER   S=SNACKS   E=EXERCISE

HOW I FEEL

😃 😊 😐 ☹️
○ ○ ○ ○

MO TU WE TH FR SA SU

DATE ....

DAY (64)

BREAKFAST	LUNCH	DINNER
....	....	....
....	....	....
....	....	....
....	....	....
....	....	....

SNACKS

....	....	....
....	....	....
....	....	....

TOTAL CALORIES

===================

OTHER

WEIGHT   SLEEP   WATER   PROTEIN

....

EXERCISE / OTHER ACTIVITIES   SET / REPS / DISTANCE   TIME

EXERCISE / OTHER ACTIVITIES	SET / REPS / DISTANCE	TIME
....	....	....
....	....	....
....	....	....
....	....	....

NOTES

....

....

....

6A   7   8   9   10   11   12P   1   2   3   4   5   6   7   8   9   10+

B=BREAKFAST   L=LUNCH   D=DINNER   S=SNACKS   E=EXERCISE

DAY (65)

MO TU WE TH FR SA SU

DATE ....

HOW I FEEL

😀 ○   🙂 ○   😐 ○   🙁 ○

BREAKFAST

....
....
....
....
....

SNACKS

....
....
....

LUNCH

....
....
....
....
....
....
....
....
....
....
....

DINNER

....
....
....
....
....
....
....
....

TOTAL CALORIES

WEIGHT   SLEEP   WATER   PROTEIN

OTHER

....

❤ EXERCISE / OTHER ACTIVITIES

SET / REPS / DISTANCE   TIME

.... | .... | ....
.... | .... | ....
.... | .... | ....
.... | .... | ....
.... | .... | ....

NOTES

....
....
....

🕐 6A 7 8 9 10 11 12P 1 2 3 4 5 6 7 8 9 10+

B=BREAKFAST L=LUNCH D=DINNER S=SNACKS E=EXERCISE

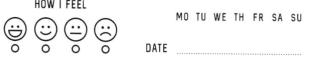

HOW I FEEL

😃 🙂 😐 🙁
○   ○   ○   ○

MO TU WE TH FR SA SU

DATE ....

DAY (66)

BREAKFAST

....
....
....
....
....
_____ ____

SNACKS

....
....
....
....

TOTAL CALORIES

_____ ____
_____

OTHER

....

LUNCH

....
....
....
....
....
....
....
....
....
....

DINNER

....
....
....
....
....
....
....
....

WEIGHT   SLEEP   WATER   PROTEIN

....

❤ EXERCISE / OTHER ACTIVITIES   SET / REPS / DISTANCE   TIME

....
....
....
....
....

NOTES

....
....
....

🕐 6A 7 8 9 10 11 12P 1 2 3 4 5 6 7 8 9 10+

B=BREAKFAST   L=LUNCH   D=DINNER   S=SNACKS   E=EXERCISE

DAY (67)

MO TU WE TH FR SA SU

DATE ....

HOW I FEEL

☺ ☺ ☺ ☹
○ ○ ○ ○

BREAKFAST

....
....
....
....
....

SNACKS

....
....
....

TOTAL CALORIES

OTHER

....

LUNCH

....
....
....
....
....
....
....
....
....
....

DINNER

....
....
....
....
....
....
....
....
....

WEIGHT   **SLEEP**   **WATER**   **PROTEIN**

....

EXERCISE / OTHER ACTIVITIES

	SET / REPS / DISTANCE	TIME
....	....	....
....	....	....
....	....	....
....	....	....
....	....	....

NOTES

....
....
....

6A 7 8 9 10 11 12P 1 2 3 4 5 6 7 8 9 10+

B=BREAKFAST L=LUNCH D=DINNER S=SNACKS E=EXERCISE

HOW I FEEL

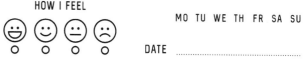

MO TU WE TH FR SA SU

DATE ....

DAY (68)

BREAKFAST

....
....
....
....
....
_____

SNACKS

....
....
....
_____

TOTAL CALORIES

_____

OTHER

....

LUNCH

....
....
....
....
....
....
....
....
....
....
_____

DINNER

....
....
....
....
_____

WEIGHT **SLEEP** **WATER** **PROTEIN**

....

EXERCISE / OTHER ACTIVITIES

	SET / REPS / DISTANCE	TIME
....	....	....
....	....	....
....	....	....
....	....	....
_____	_____	_____

NOTES

....
....
....

6A 7 8 9 10 11 12P 1 2 3 4 5 6 7 8 9 10+

B=BREAKFAST L=LUNCH D=DINNER S=SNACKS E=EXERCISE

DAY (69)

DATE ....

HOW I FEEL

😃 ☺ 😐 ☹
○ ○ ○ ○

BREAKFAST	LUNCH	DINNER
....	....	....
....	....	....
....	....	....
....	....	....
....	....	....

SNACKS

....
....
....
....

TOTAL CALORIES

_____

WEIGHT   SLEEP   WATER   PROTEIN

OTHER

....

EXERCISE / OTHER ACTIVITIES	SET / REPS / DISTANCE	TIME
....	....	....
....	....	....
....	....	....
....	....	....
....	....	....

NOTES

....
....
....

6A 7 8 9 10 11 12P 1 2 3 4 5 6 7 8 9 10+
B=BREAKFAST   L=LUNCH   D=DINNER   S=SNACKS   E=EXERCISE

HOW I FEEL

😃 ○   🙂 ○   😐 ○   🙁 ○

MO TU WE TH FR SA SU

DATE ....

DAY (70)

BREAKFAST	LUNCH	DINNER
....	....	....
....	....	....
....	....	....
....	....	....
....	....	....

SNACKS

....	....	....
....	....	....
....	....	....

TOTAL CALORIES

_____

OTHER

....

WEIGHT	SLEEP	WATER	PROTEIN

....

❤ **EXERCISE / OTHER ACTIVITIES**   SET / REPS / DISTANCE   TIME

....	....	....
....	....	....
....	....	....
....	....	....
....	....	....

NOTES

....

....

....

 6A 7 8 9 10 11 12P 1 2 3 4 5 6 7 8 9 10+

B=BREAKFAST L=LUNCH D=DINNER S=SNACKS E=EXERCISE

DAY (71)

HOW I FEEL

☺ ☺ ☺ ☹
○   ○   ○   ○

BREAKFAST   LUNCH   DINNER

....
....
....
....
....

SNACKS   ....
....
....
....

TOTAL CALORIES

WEIGHT   SLEEP   WATER   PROTEIN

OTHER
....

EXERCISE / OTHER ACTIVITIES   SET / REPS / DISTANCE   TIME

....
....
....
....
....

NOTES
....
....
....

6A 7 8 9 10 11 12P 1 2 3 4 5 6 7 8 9 10+

B=BREAKFAST   L=LUNCH   D=DINNER   S=SNACKS   E=EXERCISE

HOW I FEEL

MO TU WE TH FR SA SU

DATE ....

DAY (72)

BREAKFAST   LUNCH   DINNER

....
....
....
....
....

SNACKS   ....
....
....
....

TOTAL CALORIES   WEIGHT   SLEEP   WATER   PROTEIN

OTHER
....

♥ EXERCISE / OTHER ACTIVITIES   SET / REPS / DISTANCE   TIME

....
....
....
....
....

NOTES
....
....
....

🕐 6A 7   8   9   10   11   12P   1   2   3   4   5   6   7   8   9   10+
    B=BREAKFAST   L=LUNCH   D=DINNER   S=SNACKS   E=EXERCISE

DAY (73)

MO TU WE TH FR SA SU

DATE ....

HOW I FEEL

BREAKFAST   LUNCH   DINNER

....
....
....
....
....

SNACKS   ....

....
....
....

TOTAL CALORIES

                         WEIGHT   SLEEP   WATER   PROTEIN
OTHER

....

EXERCISE / OTHER ACTIVITIES   SET / REPS / DISTANCE   TIME

....
....
....
....
....

NOTES

....
....
....

6A 7 8 9 10 11 12P 1 2 3 4 5 6 7 8 9 10+

B=BREAKFAST L=LUNCH D=DINNER S=SNACKS E=EXERCISE

HOW I FEEL

☺ ☺ ☺ ☹
○ ○ ○ ○

MO TU WE TH FR SA SU

DATE ....

DAY (74)

BREAKFAST

....
....
....
....
....
_____ __

SNACKS

....
....
....

TOTAL CALORIES

═══════════════

OTHER

....

LUNCH

....
....
....
....
....
....
....
....
....
....

DINNER

....
....
....
....
....
....
....
....

WEIGHT   **SLEEP**   **WATER**   **PROTEIN**

....

♡ EXERCISE / OTHER ACTIVITIES

SET / REPS / DISTANCE   TIME

.... | .... | ....
.... | .... | ....
.... | .... | ....
.... | .... | ....
.... | .... | ....

NOTES

....
....
....

🕐 6A 7 8 9 10 11 12P 1 2 3 4 5 6 7 8 9 10+

B=BREAKFAST   L=LUNCH   D=DINNER   S=SNACKS   E=EXERCISE

DAY (75)

MO TU WE TH FR SA SU

DATE ....

HOW I FEEL

☺ ☺ ☺ ☹
○ ○ ○ ○

BREAKFAST   LUNCH   DINNER

....
....
....
....
....

SNACKS   ....
....
....
....

TOTAL CALORIES

WEIGHT   SLEEP   WATER   PROTEIN

OTHER

....

❤ EXERCISE / OTHER ACTIVITIES   SET / REPS / DISTANCE   TIME

....
....
....
....
....

NOTES

....
....
....

6A 7 8 9 10 11 12P 1 2 3 4 5 6 7 8 9 10+

B=BREAKFAST   L=LUNCH   D=DINNER   S=SNACKS   E=EXERCISE

DAY 75

MY MEASUREMENTS

[1] NECK

[2] CHEST

[3] ARMS

[4] WAIST

[5] ABDOMEN

[6] HIPS

[7] THIGHS

[8] CALVES

WEIGHT

BMI

DAY (76)

DATE ....

HOW I FEEL

😃   🙂   😐   🙁
○   ○   ○   ○

BREAKFAST   LUNCH   DINNER

....
....
....
....
....

SNACKS
....
....
....

TOTAL CALORIES

WEIGHT   SLEEP   WATER   PROTEIN

OTHER
....

💓 EXERCISE / OTHER ACTIVITIES   SET / REPS / DISTANCE   TIME

....
....
....
....
....

NOTES
....
....
....

🕐 6A 7 8 9 10 11 12P 1 2 3 4 5 6 7 8 9 10+

B=BREAKFAST   L=LUNCH   D=DINNER   S=SNACKS   E=EXERCISE

HOW I FEEL

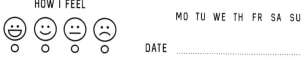

😃 😊 😐 ☹️
○ ○ ○ ○

MO TU WE TH FR SA SU

DATE ....

DAY (77)

BREAKFAST

LUNCH

DINNER

SNACKS

TOTAL CALORIES

WEIGHT   SLEEP   WATER   PROTEIN

OTHER

❤️ EXERCISE / OTHER ACTIVITIES

SET / REPS / DISTANCE   TIME

NOTES

🕐 6A 7 8 9 10 11 12P 1 2 3 4 5 6 7 8 9 10+

B=BREAKFAST L=LUNCH D=DINNER S=SNACKS E=EXERCISE

DAY (78)

DATE ....

HOW I FEEL

😃   🙂   😐   🙁
○   ○   ○   ○

BREAKFAST	LUNCH	DINNER
....	....	....
....	....	....
....	....	....
....	....	....
....	....	....

SNACKS

....	....	....
....	....	....
....	....	....

TOTAL CALORIES

WEIGHT   SLEEP   WATER   PROTEIN

OTHER

....

❤️ EXERCISE / OTHER ACTIVITIES   SET / REPS / DISTANCE   TIME

....	....	....
....	....	....
....	....	....
....	....	....
....	....	....

NOTES

....
....
....

🕐 6A 7 8 9 10 11 12P 1 2 3 4 5 6 7 8 9 10+

B=BREAKFAST   L=LUNCH   D=DINNER   S=SNACKS   E=EXERCISE

HOW I FEEL

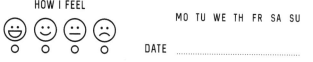

☺ ☺ ☹ ☹
○ ○ ○ ○

MO TU WE TH FR SA SU

DATE ....

DAY (79)

BREAKFAST

LUNCH

DINNER

SNACKS

TOTAL CALORIES

OTHER

WEIGHT   SLEEP   WATER   PROTEIN

EXERCISE / OTHER ACTIVITIES   SET / REPS / DISTANCE   TIME

NOTES

6A   7   8   9   10   11   12P   1   2   3   4   5   6   7   8   9   10+

B=BREAKFAST   L=LUNCH   D=DINNER   S=SNACKS   E=EXERCISE

DAY (80)

MO TU WE TH FR SA SU

DATE ....

HOW I FEEL

😃 ☺ 😐 🙁
○ ○ ○ ○

BREAKFAST	LUNCH	DINNER

SNACKS

TOTAL CALORIES

WEIGHT SLEEP WATER PROTEIN

OTHER

EXERCISE / OTHER ACTIVITIES | SET / REPS / DISTANCE | TIME

NOTES

6A 7 8 9 10 11 12P 1 2 3 4 5 6 7 8 9 10+

B=BREAKFAST L=LUNCH D=DINNER S=SNACKS E=EXERCISE

HOW I FEEL

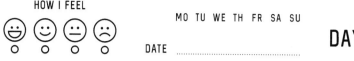

😃 😊 😐 ☹️
○ ○ ○ ○

MO TU WE TH FR SA SU

DATE ....

DAY (81)

BREAKFAST	LUNCH	DINNER
....	....	....
....	....	....
....	....	....
....	....	....
....	....	....

SNACKS

.... | .... | ....
.... | .... | ....
.... | .... | ....

TOTAL CALORIES
_____

OTHER

WEIGHT   SLEEP   WATER   PROTEIN

....

❤ EXERCISE / OTHER ACTIVITIES   SET / REPS / DISTANCE   TIME

.... | .... | ....
.... | .... | ....
.... | .... | ....
.... | .... | ....

NOTES

....
....
....

🕐 6A 7 8 9 10 11 12P 1 2 3 4 5 6 7 8 9 10+

B=BREAKFAST   L=LUNCH   D=DINNER   S=SNACKS   E=EXERCISE

DAY (82)

MO TU WE TH FR SA SU

DATE ....

HOW I FEEL

😀   🙂   😐   🙁
○   ○   ○   ○

BREAKFAST

LUNCH

DINNER

SNACKS

TOTAL CALORIES

WEIGHT   SLEEP   WATER   PROTEIN

OTHER

♡ EXERCISE / OTHER ACTIVITIES   SET / REPS / DISTANCE   TIME

NOTES

🕐 6A 7 8 9 10 11 12P 1 2 3 4 5 6 7 8 9 10+

B=BREAKFAST L=LUNCH D=DINNER S=SNACKS E=EXERCISE

HOW I FEEL

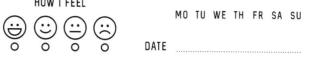

MO TU WE TH FR SA SU

DATE ....

DAY (83)

BREAKFAST   LUNCH   DINNER

SNACKS

TOTAL CALORIES

OTHER

WEIGHT   SLEEP   WATER   PROTEIN

EXERCISE / OTHER ACTIVITIES   SET / REPS / DISTANCE   TIME

NOTES

6A 7 8 9 10 11 12P 1 2 3 4 5 6 7 8 9 10+

B=BREAKFAST   L=LUNCH   D=DINNER   S=SNACKS   E=EXERCISE

DAY (84)

DATE ....

HOW I FEEL

😃 🙂 😐 🙁
○ ○ ○ ○

BREAKFAST	LUNCH	DINNER
....	....	....
....	....	....
....	....	....
....	....	....
....	....	....
	....	....

SNACKS

....

....

....

TOTAL CALORIES

_____

OTHER

....

WEIGHT	SLEEP	WATER	PROTEIN

....

❤ EXERCISE / OTHER ACTIVITIES   SET / REPS / DISTANCE   TIME

	SET / REPS / DISTANCE	TIME
....	....	....
....	....	....
....	....	....
....	....	....
....	....	....

NOTES

....

....

....

🕐 6A 7 8 9 10 11 12P 1 2 3 4 5 6 7 8 9 10+

B=BREAKFAST   L=LUNCH   D=DINNER   S=SNACKS   E=EXERCISE

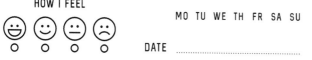

HOW I FEEL

😄 ◯ 🙂 ◯ 😐 ◯ ☹ ◯

MO TU WE TH FR SA SU

DATE ....

DAY (85)

BREAKFAST   LUNCH   DINNER

....
....
....
....
....
_____   __   ....

SNACKS   ....
....
....
....

TOTAL CALORIES
_____   WEIGHT   SLEEP   WATER   PROTEIN
OTHER
....

EXERCISE / OTHER ACTIVITIES   SET / REPS / DISTANCE   TIME

....
....
....
....
_____   _____   _____

NOTES
....
....
....

6A 7 8 9 10 11 12P 1 2 3 4 5 6 7 8 9 10+
B=BREAKFAST L=LUNCH D=DINNER S=SNACKS E=EXERCISE

DAY (86)

MO TU WE TH FR SA SU

DATE ....

HOW I FEEL

:D :) :| :(
o   o   o   o

BREAKFAST   LUNCH   DINNER

....
....
....
....
....

SNACKS   ....
....
....
....

TOTAL CALORIES

WEIGHT   SLEEP   WATER   PROTEIN

OTHER

....

EXERCISE / OTHER ACTIVITIES   SET / REPS / DISTANCE   TIME

....
....
....
....
....

NOTES

....
....
....

6A 7 8 9 10 11 12P 1 2 3 4 5 6 7 8 9 10+

B=BREAKFAST L=LUNCH D=DINNER S=SNACKS E=EXERCISE

HOW I FEEL

MO TU WE TH FR SA SU

DATE ....

DAY (87)

BREAKFAST   LUNCH   DINNER

....
....
....
....
....
_____   ....
                       ....
SNACKS   ....
....
....
....
_____   ....   _____

TOTAL CALORIES

_____   WEIGHT   SLEEP   WATER   PROTEIN

OTHER
....

EXERCISE / OTHER ACTIVITIES   SET / REPS / DISTANCE   TIME

....
....
....
....
....
_____

NOTES
....
....
....

6A 7   8   9   10 11 12P 1   2   3   4   5   6   7   8   9   10+
B=BREAKFAST   L=LUNCH   D=DINNER   S=SNACKS   E=EXERCISE

DAY (88)

MO TU WE TH FR SA SU

DATE ....

HOW I FEEL

:D :) :| :(
o   o   o   o

BREAKFAST   LUNCH   DINNER

SNACKS

TOTAL CALORIES

WEIGHT   SLEEP   WATER   PROTEIN

OTHER

EXERCISE / OTHER ACTIVITIES   SET / REPS / DISTANCE   TIME

NOTES

6A 7 8 9 10 11 12P 1 2 3 4 5 6 7 8 9 10+

B=BREAKFAST L=LUNCH D=DINNER S=SNACKS E=EXERCISE

HOW I FEEL

MO TU WE TH FR SA SU

DATE ....

DAY (89)

BREAKFAST

LUNCH

DINNER

SNACKS

TOTAL CALORIES

OTHER

WEIGHT   SLEEP   WATER   PROTEIN

 EXERCISE / OTHER ACTIVITIES   SET / REPS / DISTANCE   TIME

NOTES

6A   7   8   9   10   11   12P   1   2   3   4   5   6   7   8   9   10+

B=BREAKFAST   L=LUNCH   D=DINNER   S=SNACKS   E=EXERCISE

DAY (90)

MO TU WE TH FR SA SU

DATE ....

HOW I FEEL

😃 ☺ 😐 ☹
○ ○ ○ ○

BREAKFAST .... LUNCH .... DINNER

....
....
....
....
....

SNACKS

....
....
....

TOTAL CALORIES

WEIGHT .... SLEEP .... WATER .... PROTEIN

OTHER

....

💓 EXERCISE / OTHER ACTIVITIES .... SET / REPS / DISTANCE .... TIME

....
....
....
....
....

NOTES

....
....
....

🕐 6A 7 8 9 10 11 12P 1 2 3 4 5 6 7 8 9 10+

B=BREAKFAST L=LUNCH D=DINNER S=SNACKS E=EXERCISE

HOW I FEEL

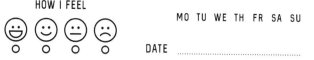

MO TU WE TH FR SA SU

DATE ....

DAY (91)

BREAKFAST   LUNCH   DINNER
....
....
....
....
....

SNACKS   ....
....
....
....

TOTAL CALORIES

WEIGHT   SLEEP   WATER   PROTEIN

OTHER
....

EXERCISE / OTHER ACTIVITIES   SET / REPS / DISTANCE   TIME
....
....
....
....
....

NOTES
....
....
....

6A 7 8 9 10 11 12P 1 2 3 4 5 6 7 8 9 10+
B=BREAKFAST L=LUNCH D=DINNER S=SNACKS E=EXERCISE

DAY (92)

MO TU WE TH FR SA SU

DATE ....

HOW I FEEL

BREAKFAST   LUNCH   DINNER

....
....
....
....
....

SNACKS   ....
....
....
....

TOTAL CALORIES

WEIGHT   SLEEP   WATER   PROTEIN

OTHER

....

EXERCISE / OTHER ACTIVITIES   SET / REPS / DISTANCE   TIME

NOTES

6A 7 8 9 10 11 12P 1 2 3 4 5 6 7 8 9 10+

B=BREAKFAST   L=LUNCH   D=DINNER   S=SNACKS   E=EXERCISE

HOW I FEEL

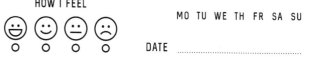

MO TU WE TH FR SA SU

DATE ....

DAY (93)

BREAKFAST	LUNCH	DINNER
....	....	....
....	....	....
....	....	....
....	....	....
....	....	....

SNACKS

TOTAL CALORIES

WEIGHT   SLEEP   WATER   PROTEIN

OTHER

....

❤ EXERCISE / OTHER ACTIVITIES

SET / REPS / DISTANCE   TIME

NOTES

6A 7 8 9 10 11 12P 1 2 3 4 5 6 7 8 9 10+

B=BREAKFAST   L=LUNCH   D=DINNER   S=SNACKS   E=EXERCISE

DAY (94)

DATE ....

HOW I FEEL

😃 😊 😐 ☹️
○ ○ ○ ○

BREAKFAST   LUNCH   DINNER

....
....
....
....
....

SNACKS   ....

....
....
....

TOTAL CALORIES

_____   WEIGHT   SLEEP   WATER   PROTEIN

OTHER

....

❤️ EXERCISE / OTHER ACTIVITIES   SET / REPS / DISTANCE   TIME

....
....
....
....
....

NOTES

....
....
....

🕐 6A 7 8 9 10 11 12P 1 2 3 4 5 6 7 8 9 10+

B=BREAKFAST   L=LUNCH   D=DINNER   S=SNACKS   E=EXERCISE

HOW I FEEL

:smile: :slight_smile: :neutral: :frowning:
O O O O

MO TU WE TH FR SA SU

DATE ....

DAY (95)

BREAKFAST	LUNCH	DINNER
....	....	....
....	....	....
....	....	....
....	....	....
....	....	....

SNACKS
....
....
....

TOTAL CALORIES
_____

OTHER

WEIGHT   SLEEP   WATER   PROTEIN

....

:heart: EXERCISE / OTHER ACTIVITIES   SET / REPS / DISTANCE   TIME

EXERCISE / OTHER ACTIVITIES	SET / REPS / DISTANCE	TIME
....	....	....
....	....	....
....	....	....
....	....	....
....	....	....

NOTES
....
....
....

6A   7   8   9   10   11   12P   1   2   3   4   5   6   7   8   9   10+

B=BREAKFAST   L=LUNCH   D=DINNER   S=SNACKS   E=EXERCISE

DAY (96)

MO TU WE TH FR SA SU

DATE ....

HOW I FEEL

BREAKFAST   LUNCH   DINNER

SNACKS

TOTAL CALORIES

WEIGHT   SLEEP   WATER   PROTEIN

OTHER

EXERCISE / OTHER ACTIVITIES   SET / REPS / DISTANCE   TIME

NOTES

6A 7 8 9 10 11 12P 1 2 3 4 5 6 7 8 9 10+

B=BREAKFAST   L=LUNCH   D=DINNER   S=SNACKS   E=EXERCISE

HOW I FEEL

MO TU WE TH FR SA SU

DATE ....

DAY (97)

BREAKFAST | LUNCH | DINNER

SNACKS

TOTAL CALORIES

WEIGHT   SLEEP   WATER   PROTEIN

OTHER

❤ EXERCISE / OTHER ACTIVITIES   SET / REPS / DISTANCE   TIME

NOTES

6A 7 8 9 10 11 12P 1 2 3 4 5 6 7 8 9 10+

B=BREAKFAST L=LUNCH D=DINNER S=SNACKS E=EXERCISE

DAY (98)

MO TU WE TH FR SA SU

DATE ....

HOW I FEEL

😀 😊 😐 ☹️
○ ○ ○ ○

BREAKFAST

LUNCH

DINNER

SNACKS

TOTAL CALORIES

WEIGHT   SLEEP   WATER   PROTEIN

OTHER

EXERCISE / OTHER ACTIVITIES   SET / REPS / DISTANCE   TIME

NOTES

6A 7 8 9 10 11 12P 1 2 3 4 5 6 7 8 9 10+

B=BREAKFAST   L=LUNCH   D=DINNER   S=SNACKS   E=EXERCISE

HOW I FEEL

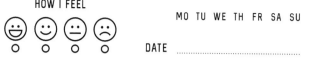

😃 🙂 😐 ☹️
○ ○ ○ ○

MO TU WE TH FR SA SU

DATE ....

DAY (99)

BREAKFAST   LUNCH   DINNER

....
....
....
....
....

SNACKS

....
....
....

TOTAL CALORIES

═══════════════

OTHER   WEIGHT   SLEEP   WATER   PROTEIN

....

EXERCISE / OTHER ACTIVITIES   SET / REPS / DISTANCE   TIME

....
....
....
....
....

NOTES

....
....
....

6A 7 8 9 10 11 12P 1 2 3 4 5 6 7 8 9 10+

B=BREAKFAST L=LUNCH D=DINNER S=SNACKS E=EXERCISE

DAY (100)

DATE ....

HOW I FEEL

☺ ☺ 😐 ☹
○ ○ ○ ○

BREAKFAST | LUNCH | DINNER

....
....
....
....
....

SNACKS

....
....
....

TOTAL CALORIES

WEIGHT   SLEEP   WATER   PROTEIN

OTHER

....

❤ EXERCISE / OTHER ACTIVITIES   SET / REPS / DISTANCE   TIME

....
....
....
....
....

NOTES

....
....
....

6A 7 8 9 10 11 12P 1 2 3 4 5 6 7 8 9 10+

B=BREAKFAST   L=LUNCH   D=DINNER   S=SNACKS   E=EXERCISE

DAY 100

MY MEASUREMENTS

[1] NECK

[2] CHEST

[3] ARMS

[4] WAIST

[5] ABDOMEN

[6] HIPS

[7] THIGHS

[8] CALVES

BMI

WEIGHT

MY RESULTS

DAY **1**   DAY **100**

BEFORE	AFTER	DIFFERENCE
....	....	[1] NECK
....	....	[2] CHEST
....	....	[3] ARMS
....	....	[4] WAIST
....	....	[5] ABDOMEN
....	....	[6] HIPS
....	....	[7] THIGHS
....	....	[8] CALVES

WEIGHT   WEIGHT   WEIGHT

BMI   BMI   BMI

NOTES

....

....

....

....

....

....

....

....

....

....

....

....

....

....

....

....

....

....

....

....

....

COPYRIGHT © GET FIT NOTEBOOKS
PUBLISHED BY: STUDIO 5519, 1732 1ST AVE #25519 NEW YORK, NY 10128
APRIL 2017, ISSUE NO. 1 [V 1.0]: CONTACT: INFO@STUDIO5519.COM; ILLUSTRATION CREDITS: © DEPOSITPHOTOS / @ PUSHINKA11

Made in the USA
Middletown, DE
28 October 2017